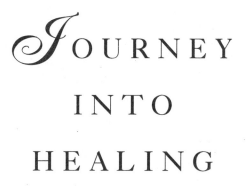

JOURNEY
INTO
HEALING

Other books by Deepak Chopra, M.D.

CREATING HEALTH

RETURN OF THE RISHI

QUANTUM HEALING

PERFECT HEALTH

UNCONDITIONAL LIFE

AGELESS BODY, TIMELESS MIND

CREATING AFFLUENCE

PERFECT WEIGHT

RESTFUL SLEEP

JOURNEY INTO HEALING

AWAKENING THE
WISDOM WITHIN YOU

• • •

DEEPAK CHOPRA, M.D.

• • •

HARMONY BOOKS • NEW YORK

Published by Harmony Books, a division of Crown Publishers, Inc., 201 East 50th Street, New York, New York 10022. Member of the Crown Publishing Group.

Random House, Inc. New York, Toronto, London, Sydney, Auckland

HARMONY and colophon are trademarks of Crown Publishers, Inc.

Manufactured in the United States of America

Library of Congress Cataloging-in-Publication Data

Chopra, Deepak
Journey into healing : awakening the wisdom within you—1st ed.
1. Healing—Quotations, maxims, etc. I. Title.
RZ999.C444   1994
610—dc20   94-20937

ISBN 0-517-79973-1
10 9 8 7 6 5 4 3 2 1
First Edition

My special gratitude to
Henry Bloomstein for his skillful
assistance in compiling the
selections for this book.

*I*nsights are inner visions and they change our lives. The cosmic mind whispers to us in the silent spaces between our thoughts and there is a sudden knowingness and we are transformed. Insights are mutations in consciousness that can radically change our physical bodies and alter our experiences of the world. When a flash of insight first comes, it is not verbal, not linguistically structured—it is a feeling of sudden knowledge and it is liberating, because without words we know it as truth. Later, this knowledge is put into words and the words reinforce the knowingness that has already occurred. I hope the words expressed in the following pages will remind you of the truth that is already known to you.

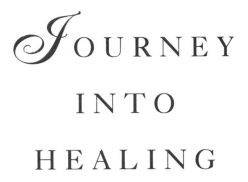

JOURNEY

INTO

HEALING

I

Perfect health, pure
and invincible, is a state we have
lost. Regain it, and we regain
a world.

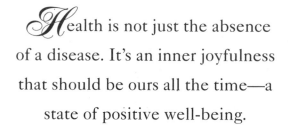

Health is not just the absence of a disease. It's an inner joyfulness that should be ours all the time—a state of positive well-being.

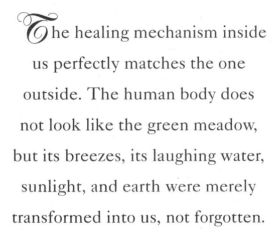

The healing mechanism inside us perfectly matches the one outside. The human body does not look like the green meadow, but its breezes, its laughing water, sunlight, and earth were merely transformed into us, not forgotten.

We all need to be healed in the highest sense by making ourselves perfect in mind, body, and spirit. The first step is to realize that this is even possible.

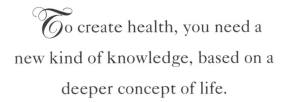

To create health, you need a
new kind of knowledge, based on a
deeper concept of life.

Although our package
of skin and bones looks very
convincing, it is a mask, an
illusion, disguising our true self,
which has no limitations.

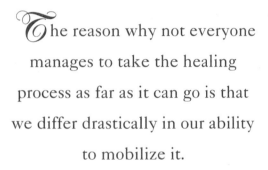

The reason why not everyone manages to take the healing process as far as it can go is that we differ drastically in our ability to mobilize it.

There are some things that require no work, and healing is one of them. You don't have to work to achieve a silent mind; you don't have to work to find the old wounds. All these things are a given, once they are uncovered. The uncovering begins wherever you are now, but its goal is always the same—the revelation of wholeness that unites body, mind, and spirit as one.

II

Health and disease are
connected like variations on one
melody. But disease is a wrong
variation, a distortion of
that theme.

The cause of disease is often extremely complex, but one thing can be said for certain: no one has proved that getting sick is necessary.

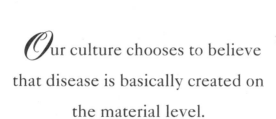

*O*ur culture chooses to believe
that disease is basically created on
the material level.

Matter is a captive moment in space and time, and by seeing our world and the universe materialistically, we make the captive aspects of the universe assume too much importance.

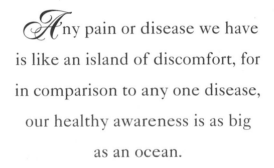

*A*ny pain or disease we have
is like an island of discomfort, for
in comparison to any one disease,
our healthy awareness is as big
as an ocean.

*I*n a serious or life-threatening illness, there can be many layers of imbalance concealing the depths where healing exists.

III

To live without love, compassion, or any other spiritual value creates a state of such severe imbalance that every cell yearns to correct it. Ultimately, that is what lies behind the onset of disease: the body is sending a message that something lacking in the present—an imbalance existing somewhere—has given rise to highly visible, unarguable, physical symptoms.

IV

Before the art of medicine

comes the art of belief.

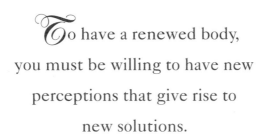

To have a renewed body,
you must be willing to have new
perceptions that give rise to
new solutions.

We are the only creatures on
earth who can change our biology
by what we think and feel.

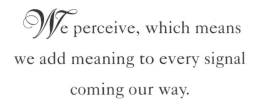

We perceive, which means
we add meaning to every signal
coming our way.

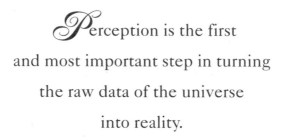

*P*erception is the first
and most important step in turning
the raw data of the universe
into reality.

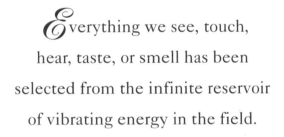

*E*verything we see, touch,
hear, taste, or smell has been
selected from the infinite reservoir
of vibrating energy in the field.

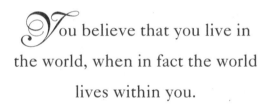

$\mathcal{Y}$ou believe that you live in
the world, when in fact the world
lives within you.

I recall the fascinating sight of a beekeeper who reached into the swarm of bees, and by gently unfolding the queen in his hands, moved the whole hive—a living globe of insects suspended in midair. What was he moving? There was no solid mass, only an image of hovering, darting, ever-changing life centered around a single focal point. The swarm is an illusion of shape behind which the reality is pure change. Such are we too. We are a swarm of molecules hovering around an invisible center.

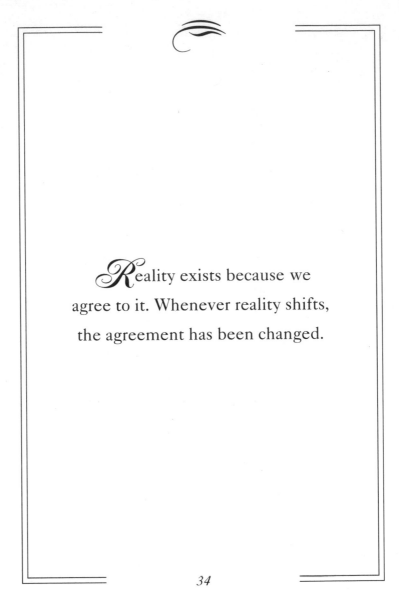

$\mathcal{R}$eality exists because we
agree to it. Whenever reality shifts,
the agreement has been changed.

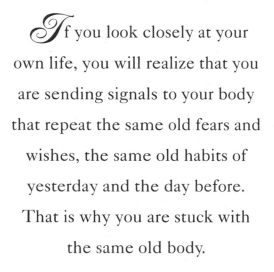

*I*f you look closely at your own life, you will realize that you are sending signals to your body that repeat the same old fears and wishes, the same old habits of yesterday and the day before. That is why you are stuck with the same old body.

The point that Archimedes was looking for—a place to stand on and move the world—actually exists. It is inside us, covered up by the fascinating but misleading moving-picture show of the waking state.

We all create scenarios
and then become convinced by
them, down to our very cells.

$\mathcal{B}$ad habits are just the
worn-out ruts of the mind, paths
that once led to freedom because
they opened up new thoughts, but
now lead nowhere.

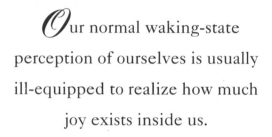

*O*ur normal waking-state
perception of ourselves is usually
ill-equipped to realize how much
joy exists inside us.

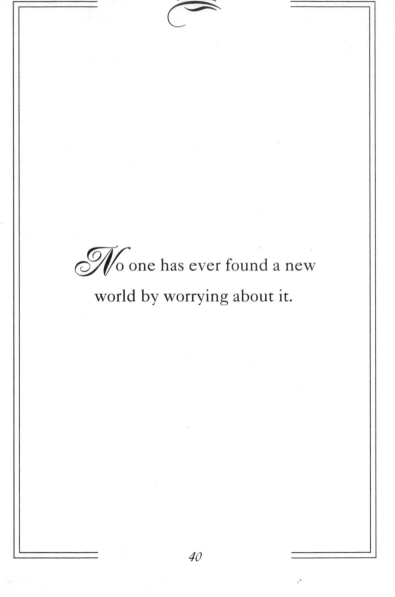

No one has ever found a new

world by worrying about it.

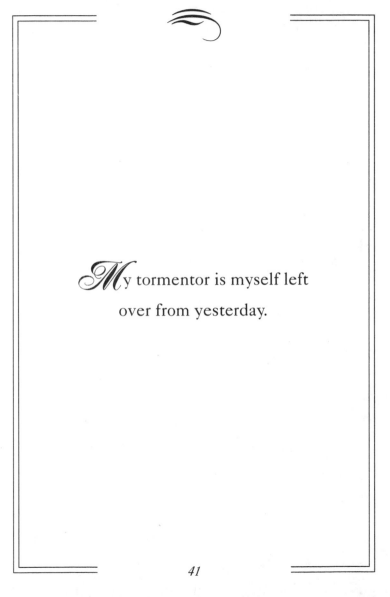

My tormentor is myself left

over from yesterday.

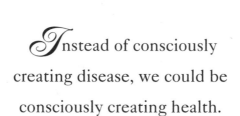

$\mathcal{I}$nstead of consciously
creating disease, we could be
consciously creating health.

$\mathcal{W}$hen you realize that you have
control over any interpretation
you place upon your body, an
enormously liberating idea begins
to dawn: the body is on your side.

$\mathcal{O}$ur essential state is that we are

completely dimensionless—pure

potentiality that can manifest into

any form, into any phenomena

in creation.

We all have the power to
make reality. Why make it inside
boundaries when the boundless
is so near?

$\mathcal{M}$y hard belief that life
is merciless, like a mill wheel
impartially grinding out birth and
death, is gone. To see things that
way is to accept the appearance
and miss the essence. Come closer,
and the world looks much more
like a wish, a great desire coming
true all around us, with our own
wishes and desires woven into it.

V

*M*atter and energy come
and go, flickering in and out of
existence like fireflies, yet all
events are held together and made
orderly by the deep intelligence
that runs through all things.

*O*nce you agree that your
self is intelligent, then all creating
is within your grasp through the
principle of self-referral:
"Curving back within myself, I
create again and again," as the
Bhagavad Gita says.

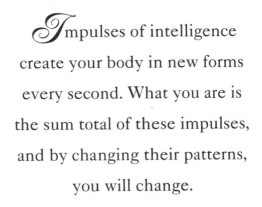

$\mathcal{I}$mpulses of intelligence create your body in new forms every second. What you are is the sum total of these impulses, and by changing their patterns, you will change.

$\mathcal{N}$o matter how different they
appear, body and mind are both
soaked through with intelligence.

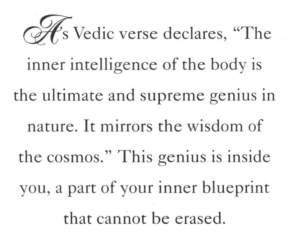

$\mathscr{A}$s Vedic verse declares, "The inner intelligence of the body is the ultimate and supreme genius in nature. It mirrors the wisdom of the cosmos." This genius is inside you, a part of your inner blueprint that cannot be erased.

*E*very cell is a miniature
terminal connected to the cosmic
computer.

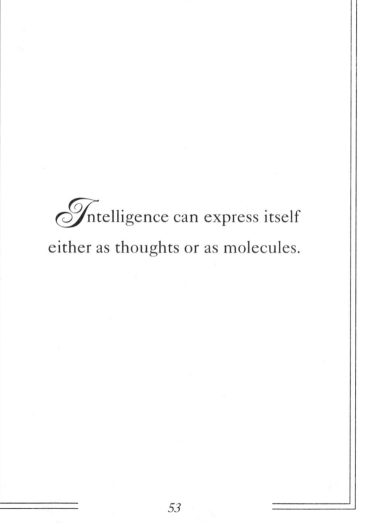

*I*ntelligence can express itself
either as thoughts or as molecules.

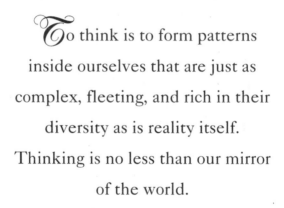

To think is to form patterns inside ourselves that are just as complex, fleeting, and rich in their diversity as is reality itself. Thinking is no less than our mirror of the world.

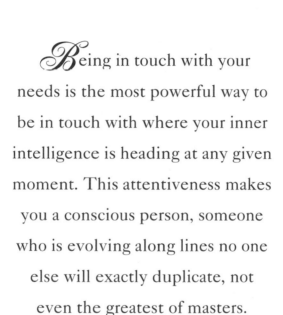

$\mathcal{B}$eing in touch with your
needs is the most powerful way to
be in touch with where your inner
intelligence is heading at any given
moment. This attentiveness makes
you a conscious person, someone
who is evolving along lines no one
else will exactly duplicate, not
even the greatest of masters.

Where Nature goes to create
stars, galaxies, quarks, and leptons,
you and I go to create ourselves.

VI

As you see it right now,

your body is the physical picture,

in 3-D, of what you are thinking.

The body is not a
frozen sculpture. It is a river of
information—a flowing organism
empowered by millions of years of
intelligence.

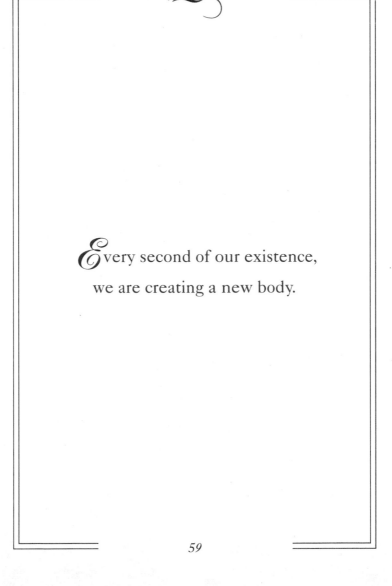

*E*very second of our existence,

we are creating a new body.

*J*ust one year ago,
98 percent of the atoms in our
bodies were not there. It's as
if we live inside buildings whose
bricks are being systematically
taken out and replaced.

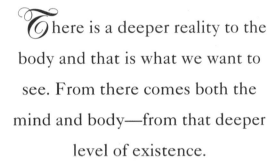

There is a deeper reality to the body and that is what we want to see. From there comes both the mind and body—from that deeper level of existence.

The human body first
takes form as intense but invisible
vibrations, called quantum
fluctuations, before it proceeds to
coalesce into impulses of energy
and particles of matter.

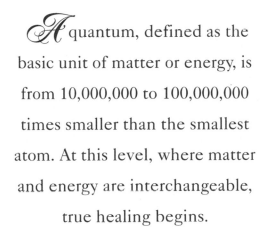

A quantum, defined as the basic unit of matter or energy, is from 10,000,000 to 100,000,000 times smaller than the smallest atom. At this level, where matter and energy are interchangeable, true healing begins.

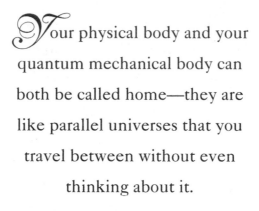

$\mathcal{Y}$our physical body and your quantum mechanical body can both be called home—they are like parallel universes that you travel between without even thinking about it.

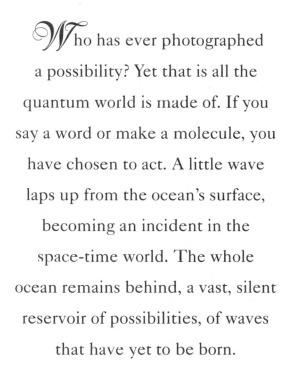

*W*ho has ever photographed
a possibility? Yet that is all the
quantum world is made of. If you
say a word or make a molecule, you
have chosen to act. A little wave
laps up from the ocean's surface,
becoming an incident in the
space-time world. The whole
ocean remains behind, a vast, silent
reservoir of possibilities, of waves
that have yet to be born.

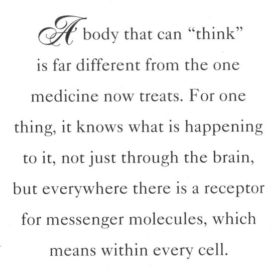

$\mathcal{A}$ body that can "think"
is far different from the one
medicine now treats. For one
thing, it knows what is happening
to it, not just through the brain,
but everywhere there is a receptor
for messenger molecules, which
means within every cell.

When you say, "I have a gut
feeling about such and such,"
you're not speaking metaphorically,
you're speaking literally, because
your gut makes the same chemicals
as your brain when it thinks.

*A*ny cell, tissue, or organ is
capable of crying out for attention,
and when you give it some, the
healing process begins.

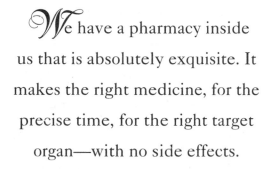

$\mathscr{W}$e have a pharmacy inside us that is absolutely exquisite. It makes the right medicine, for the precise time, for the right target organ—with no side effects.

The human body keeps in balance through complex rhythms and cycles. These biorhythms are our connecting link to the larger rhythms of Nature: the immensely long life cycles of the stars, the ebb and flow of the earth's seas, and the breathing of all living things.

$\mathscr{A}$s you cross from the ordinary waking state to higher states of awareness, the body serves as your vehicle; it is not a leaky boat you hope will get you there before you sink. But when you are truly in tune with your body, it becomes a trusted teacher and a trusted guide.

VII

Science declares that we are physical machines that have somehow learned to think. Now it dawns that we are thoughts that have learned to create a physical machine.

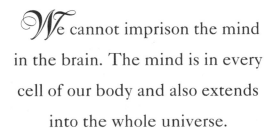

We cannot imprison the mind
in the brain. The mind is in every
cell of our body and also extends
into the whole universe.

Your mind gives you
control, the ability to have any
reaction you want.

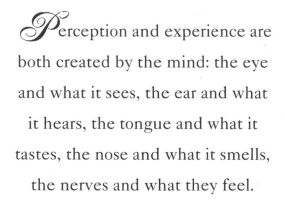

Perception and experience are both created by the mind: the eye and what it sees, the ear and what it hears, the tongue and what it tastes, the nose and what it smells, the nerves and what they feel.

$\mathcal{T}$he highest level of belief

comes when the mind contacts its

own intelligence as an experience.

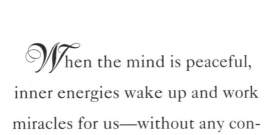

When the mind is peaceful,
inner energies wake up and work
miracles for us—without any conscious effort on our part.

In *Siddhartha*, Hermann Hesse writes, "Within you there is a stillness and sanctuary to which you can retreat at any time and be yourself." This sanctuary is a simple awareness of comfort, which can't be violated by the turmoil of events. This place feels no trauma and stores no hurt. It is the healing mental space that one seeks to find in meditation.

A quiet mind is all you need.

VIII

*B*ecause we can change like
quicksilver, the flowing quality
of life is natural to us. The
material body is a river of atoms,
the mind is a river of thought,
and what holds them together is
a river of intelligence.

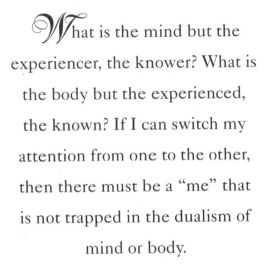

What is the mind but the experiencer, the knower? What is the body but the experienced, the known? If I can switch my attention from one to the other, then there must be a "me" that is not trapped in the dualism of mind or body.

We are not the body. We are not the mind. We are the ones who have mind and body.

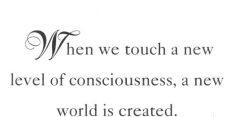

When we touch a new
level of consciousness, a new
world is created.

$\mathcal{C}$onsciousness is nothing but
awareness—the composite of all
the things we pay attention to.

The biochemistry of the body is
the product of awareness. Beliefs,
thoughts, and emotions create
the chemical reactions that uphold
life in every cell.

When we don't maintain the continuity of our awareness, all of us fall into gaps of one kind or another. Vast areas of our bodily existence go out of control, leading to sickness, aging, and death.

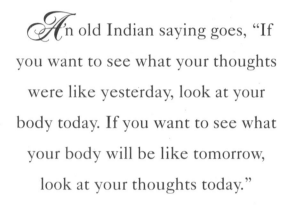

An old Indian saying goes, "If you want to see what your thoughts were like yesterday, look at your body today. If you want to see what your body will be like tomorrow, look at your thoughts today."

*H*ow infinitely beautiful the immune system is and how terribly vulnerable at the same time. It forges our link with life and yet can break it at any moment. The immune system knows all our secrets, all our sorrows. It knows why a mother who has lost a child can die of grief, because the immune system has died of grief first. It knows every moment a cancer patient spends in the light of life or the shadow of death, because it turns those moments into the body's physical reality.

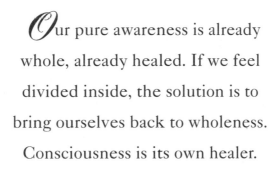

$\mathcal{O}$ur pure awareness is already whole, already healed. If we feel divided inside, the solution is to bring ourselves back to wholeness. Consciousness is its own healer.

In moments of silence,
realize that you are recontacting
your source of pure awareness.

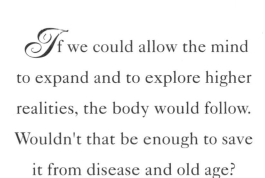

$\mathscr{I}$f we could allow the mind

to expand and to explore higher

realities, the body would follow.

Wouldn't that be enough to save

it from disease and old age?

*A*s spiritual unfoldment
becomes conscious, the circle of
life acquires another dimension.
Your sense of self expands with
no end in sight. More and more
experience is allowed to come into
the never-ending conversation that
each of us is conducting with all
50 trillion cells in our body.

IX

$\mathcal{B}$eing alive is like a wave
pulsing upward from the invisible
to the visible, from a region the
senses cannot register to one that
they can. The closer you can get to
the invisible source, the greater
your healing power.

*A*ll that is needed is to reach
the depths where transformation is
effortless and most powerful.
Our servants wait on us, but they
wait inside.

$\mathscr{A}$ shift in awareness is

the first change.

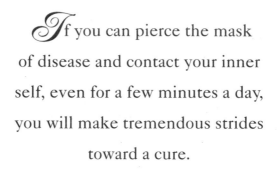

If you can pierce the mask
of disease and contact your inner
self, even for a few minutes a day,
you will make tremendous strides
toward a cure.

When we experience pure
silence in the mind, the body
becomes silent also. And in that
field of silence, healing is much
more efficient.

*Y*ou can use the quantum perspective to see your body as a silent flow of intelligence, a constant bubbling up of impulses that create, control, and become your physical body. The secret of life at this level is that *anything in your body* can be changed with the flick of an intention.

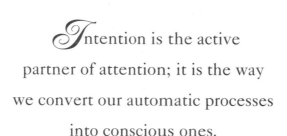

Intention is the active
partner of attention; it is the way
we convert our automatic processes
into conscious ones.

$\mathcal{W}$hen we begin to create
health, the unholy world erected
by our minds transforms itself
into a higher reality, the world of
the heart.

The so-called tender emotions
spring from the source of life;
therefore, they are incredibly
powerful.

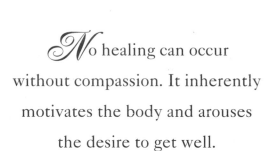

No healing can occur
without compassion. It inherently
motivates the body and arouses
the desire to get well.

At any level where emotions are allowed to touch, the current of life is restored. Nothing is mightier than that, for the current of life has borne us along, forever, safe against dangers, for billions of years of evolution. At full flood, the river of life sweeps all before it, and the most massive obstacles are pushed back into the main current like stagnant pools washed clean by the tide.

*I*n mind-body medicine,
any explanation has its roots in an
earlier stage, in the moment when
the immune system was weakened
by a negative mental influence.

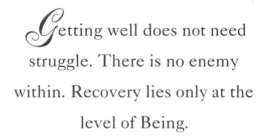

$\mathcal{G}$etting well does not need
struggle. There is no enemy
within. Recovery lies only at the
level of Being.

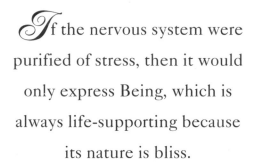

If the nervous system were purified of stress, then it would only express Being, which is always life-supporting because its nature is bliss.

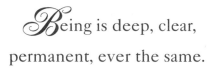

Being is deep, clear,
permanent, ever the same.

To experience bliss every hour of the day would be a sign of complete enlightenment, but even a brief encounter is significant—it permits you to actually feel waves of consciousness as they well up from the field of silence, cross the gap, and are infused into every cell. This is the body's own awakening.

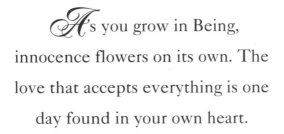

*A*s you grow in Being,
innocence flowers on its own. The
love that accepts everything is one
day found in your own heart.

When life is full, it is only love,
and when awareness is full, it
brings only love. Every impulse of
intelligence in our awareness starts
its journey from the source of life
as love, and nothing else.

The use of love is to heal.
When it flows without effort
from the depth of the self, love
creates health.

X

Understanding and experience are the two legs of healing, marching side by side. Thus the self that was crippled by fear discovers, without strain or pressure, the repressed power of truth that has been denied for so long.

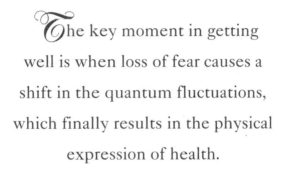

The key moment in getting well is when loss of fear causes a shift in the quantum fluctuations, which finally results in the physical expression of health.

All fear is ultimately the fear
of mortality in disguise—the fear
of change.

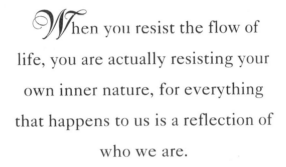

When you resist the flow of life, you are actually resisting your own inner nature, for everything that happens to us is a reflection of who we are.

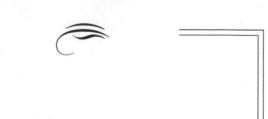

*Q*uietly, in your own heart, say
that you do not want to be afraid.

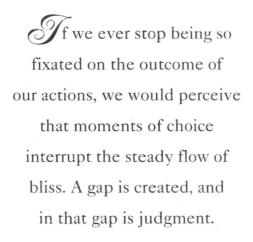

*I*f we ever stop being so
fixated on the outcome of
our actions, we would perceive
that moments of choice
interrupt the steady flow of
bliss. A gap is created, and
in that gap is judgment.

*I*ntentions automatically seek
their fulfillment if left alone.

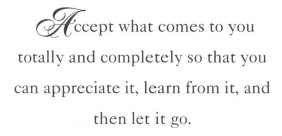

Accept what comes to you
totally and completely so that you
can appreciate it, learn from it, and
then let it go.

*I*f the body, stubborn and solid-looking as it appears, can undertake this journey, something much greater will be achieved. We will no longer just dream of freedom from the ills that flesh is heir to, we will really become free, clothed in flesh that has become as perfect as our ideals.

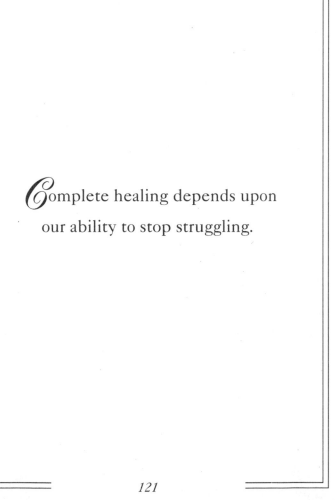

*C*omplete healing depends upon

our ability to stop struggling.

XI

To cure a disease, I have to change the cellular memory of the disease—and that comes by transcending all emotion, all thought, and by becoming the silent witness of the process.

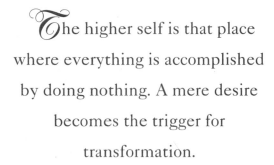

The higher self is that place where everything is accomplished by doing nothing. A mere desire becomes the trigger for transformation.

One's inner sense of "me"
is built up of images from the past,
all the fears, hopes, wishes, dreams,
loves, and disappointments one
calls "mine." However, if you
strip all these images away,
something of "me" is still left: the
decision maker, the screen, the
silent witness.

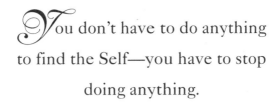

You don't have to do anything
to find the Self—you have to stop
doing anything.

When you get in touch
with the part of yourself that is
eternal and nonchanging, you have
true knowledge of your own
immortality, and fear melts away
like snow in the summer breeze.

XII

After we recover from an illness, the moment comes when the feeling of being sick gives way to being well again. "I'm a new person," you say, and you're right: your body has printed out a new creation that is healthy instead of sick.

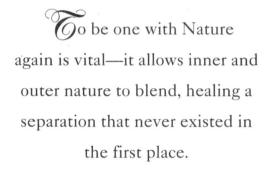

To be one with Nature
again is vital—it allows inner and
outer nature to blend, healing a
separation that never existed in
the first place.

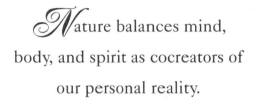

Nature balances mind,
body, and spirit as cocreators of
our personal reality.

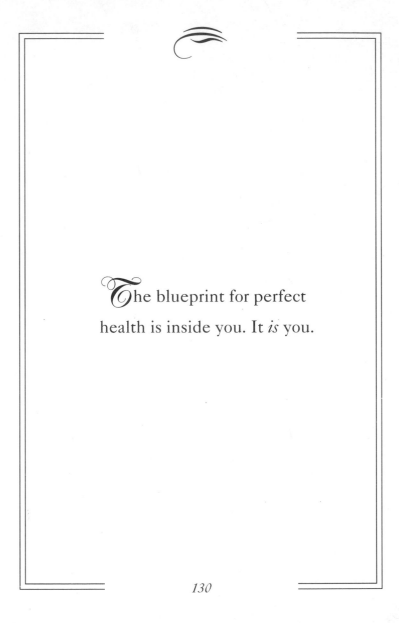

The blueprint for perfect health is inside you. It *is* you.

We are all different because we've walked through different gardens and knelt at different graves. Every little wisp of experience that has come our way we have metabolized and made into our body. And as we now go into higher states of awareness, we metabolize those experiences too. They also store the knowledge of higher realities complete and formed, and they are ready for you to unfold them.

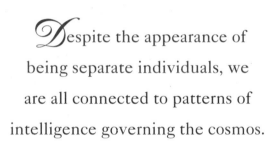

Despite the appearance of being separate individuals, we are all connected to patterns of intelligence governing the cosmos.

In ordinary waking
consciousness, you touch your
finger to a rose and feel it as solid,
but in truth one bundle of energy
and information—your finger—is
contacting another bundle of
energy and information—the rose.
Your finger and the thing it touches
are both just minute outcroppings
of the infinite field we call
the universe.

The only absolute left to us is the timeless, for now we realize that our entire universe is just one incident springing forth out of a larger reality. What we sense as seconds, minutes, hours, days, and years are cut-up bits of this larger reality.

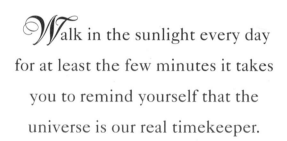

$\mathcal{W}$alk in the sunlight every day
for at least the few minutes it takes
you to remind yourself that the
universe is our real timekeeper.

*H*uman consciousness and cosmic consciousness are one. The field dances and waits for us to join it. It constantly folds and refolds itself, like an infinite wool blanket tumbling in a dryer at infinite speed.

*A*ll transformations eventually
lead back to the same source—our
own pure awareness.

An intimate relationship is one
that allows you to be yourself.

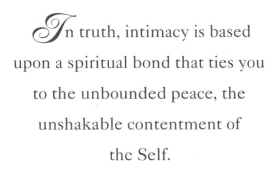

 $\mathscr{I}$ n truth, intimacy is based
upon a spiritual bond that ties you
to the unbounded peace, the
unshakable contentment of
the Self.

The deepest reality you are
aware of is the one from which you
draw your power.

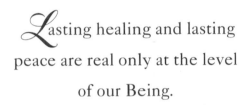

$\mathcal{L}$asting healing and lasting
peace are real only at the level
of our Being.

XIII

Healthy people live neither
in the past nor in the future. They
live in the present, in the now,
which gives the now a flavor of
eternity because no shadows
fall across it.

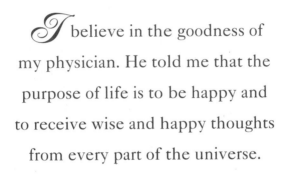

$\mathscr{I}$ believe in the goodness of
my physician. He told me that the
purpose of life is to be happy and
to receive wise and happy thoughts
from every part of the universe.

If I find a green meadow
splashed with daisies and sit down
beside a clear-running brook, I
have found medicine.

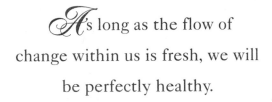

As long as the flow of
change within us is fresh, we will
be perfectly healthy.

*E*nchantment is our

natural state.

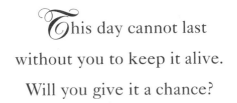

This day cannot last

without you to keep it alive.

Will you give it a chance?

*A*ttend to your own inner health and well-being. Happiness radiates like the fragrance from a flower and draws all good things toward you. Allow your love to nourish yourself as well as others. Do not strain after the needs of life—it is sufficient to be quietly alert and aware of them. In this way, life proceeds more naturally and effortlessly. Life is here to enjoy.

• • •

*I*n this book I have sought to select essential thoughts from my various books and arrange them so as to give the reader the experience of a journey into healing. I hope this journey will influence your perceptions, the better to free your body's natural tendency to perfect health. To complement this text I have added the following pages on meditation, one of the best ways to access our inner intelligence, to experience who we really are.

*A*lthough, in the west today, meditation is thought of in terms of stress management and relaxation, its true purpose is a spiritual one. The yogis and seers who first recognized these practices were already pretty relaxed living in their caves in the Himalayas. They meditated to discover their true selves; they meditated for enlightenment.

Of all the experiences we can have, the experience of our inner self is the most important. The body is the objective experience of our ideas, while the mind is the subjective experience of them. The body is ever-changing, and the mind, with its thoughts, feelings, and desires, also comes and goes. They are both experiences locked in time and space; they are not the experiencer. The one who is having the experience is beyond time and space, it is the real you. It is the timeless factor in every time-bound experience, the feeler behind the feeling, the thinker of thoughts, the animator of our bodies and minds. It is our soul.

Nowadays science has enabled us to track a thought or an intention a microsecond after it happens, but all the scientific equipment in the world still cannot tell us where the thought is coming from or who is having it. You cannot find the real you in your mind or your body because you are simply not there. We can listen to Beethoven on the radio, but there is no point in taking the radio apart to find Beethoven. He is not there. The radio is just an instrument that traps a field of information and converts it into a space-time event. Similarly, the real you is a nonlocal field of information that is trapped in space and time by the body and mind. Your soul, the thinker of thoughts, finds expression through the mind and body, but when the body and brain are destroyed, nothing happens to the real you. The unconditional spirit is not energy or matter, it is in the silent spaces between our thoughts.

There is a space between each of your thoughts where you manufacture your thoughts, where you are an infinite choice maker. This "gap" between thoughts is the window to your higher self, the window to the cosmic self. The real you cannot be squeezed into the volume of a body or the span of a lifetime. It is the thinker in the field of memory and information in the space between thoughts.

The space between thoughts is silent; it is a pregnant silence. This is a silence filled with an infinite possibility of thoughts, a field of pure potentiality.

It is the real self. The thinker is a silent, infinite choice maker that resides at the level of the "gap." The real you and the real me are both silent fields of infinite possibilities. The differences between you and me are the different possible experiences we choose at the level of the gap. Action creates memory, memory creates desire, and desire again leads to action. The seeds of our memories and desires in the gap seek manifestation through the instruments of the mind and body and create the whole world in which we live.

Our existence has three levels: (1) the physical body, made up of matter and energy; (2) the subtle body comprising the mind, intellect, and ego; and (3) the causal body, which contains the soul and the spirit. The practice of meditation takes our awareness from the disturbed state of consciousness in the mind and the world of physical objects to the silent, undisturbed state of consciousness in the realm of the soul and spirit. Through regular practice we gain access to the infinite storehouse of knowledge—the ultimate reality of creation. We have the experience of who we really are— pure unbounded consciousness. When we experience who we really are, we restore the memory of wholeness or healing in our lives.

There are many forms of meditation. The more advanced practices involve the use of mantras. Mantras are primordial sounds, the basic sounds of nature, that act as an instrument of the mind, a vehicle to take our awareness from the level of activity to the level of silence. Mantras are usually selected by a qualified instructor and taught on an individual basis. At the Center for Mind Body Medicine in San Diego we teach the Primordial Sound Meditation. Less specific but effective meditations are also available. One such practice, the Mindfulness Meditation, is described here and is an excellent way to get started.

THE MINDFULNESS MEDITATION

The Mindfulness Meditation technique is a simple meditation procedure that can create a deep state of relaxation in your mind and body. As the mind quiets down but remains awake you will experience deeper, more silent levels of awareness.

1.
Start by sitting comfortably in a quiet place where you will have a minimum amount of disturbance.

2.
Close your eyes.

3.
Breathe normally and naturally, and gently allow your awareness to be on your breathing. Simply observe your breath, trying not to control it or alter it in any conscious way.

4.

*As you observe your breath, you may notice
that it changes of its own accord. It may vary in
speed, rhythm, or depth, and there may even be
occasions when your breath seems to stop for
a time. Whatever happens with your breathing,
innocently observe it without trying to cause
or initiate any changes.*

5.

*You will find that at times your attention
drifts away from your breath and you are
thinking about other things or listening to noises
outside. Whenever you notice you are not
observing your breath, gently bring your
attention back to your breathing.*

6.

*If, during the meditation, you notice that you
are focusing on some feeling, mood, or
expectation, treat this as you would any other
thought and gently bring your attention
back to your breathing.*

7.

*Practice this meditation technique
for fifteen minutes.*

8.

*At the end of fifteen minutes, keep your eyes
closed and just sit easily for two to three minutes.
Allow yourself to come out of the meditation
gradually before opening your eyes and
resuming your activity.*

• • •

It is recommended that you practice this Mindfulness Meditation technique for about fifteen minutes twice a day in the morning and evening. You may also use this technique for a few minutes during the day to help center yourself if you are feeling upset or agitated.

• • •

During the practice of meditation you will have one of three experiences. All of these are correct experiences.

1.

You may feel bored or restless and your mind may become filled with thoughts. This is an indication that deep-rooted stresses and emotions are being released from your system. By effortlessly continuing with meditation, you will facilitate the removal of these impurities from your mind and body.

2.

You may fall asleep. If you fall asleep in meditation it is an indication that you need more rest during other times of the day.

3.

You may slip into the "gap." When the mantra or breath becomes very settled and refined, you slip into the gap between thoughts, beyond sound, beyond breath.

If you stay rested, take care of yourself, and take time to commit to meditation, you are bound to get in touch with your inner self. You will tap into the cosmic mind, the voice that whispers to you nonverbally in the silent spaces between your thoughts. This is your inner intelligence, and it is the ultimate and supreme genius that mirrors the wisdom of the universe. Trust this inner wisdom and all your dreams will come true.

•   •   •